MW00477383

5-MINUTE
GRATITUDE JOURNAL FOR MEN

Daily Prompts and Practices to Give Thanks and Practice Positivity

Scott Smith

ROCKRIDGE
PRESS

Copyright © 2022 by Rockridge Press

All rights reserved. No part of this publication may be reproduced, stored in a retrieval system, or transmitted in any form or by any means, electronic, mechanical, photocopying, recording, scanning, or otherwise without the prior written permission of the Publisher. Requests to the Publisher for permission should be addressed to the Permissions Department, Rockridge Press, 1955 Broadway, Suite 400, Oakland, CA 94612.

First Rockridge Press trade paperback edition 2022

Rockridge Press and the Rockridge Press logo are trademarks or registered trademarks of Callisto Media Inc. and/or its affiliates in the United States and other countries and may not be used without written permission.

For general information on our other products and services, please contact our Customer Care Department within the United States at (866) 744-2665, or outside the United States at (510) 253-0500.

Paperback ISBN: 978-1-68539-898-9

Manufactured in the United States of America
Interior and Cover Designer: Amanda Kirk
Art Producer: Maya Melenchuk
Editor: Owen Holmes
Production Editor: Jaime Chan
Production Manager: David Zapanta

10 9 8 7 6 5 4 3 2 1 0

This Journal Belongs To

_____

Contents

Introduction iv

How to Use This Book v

5-MINUTE JOURNAL ENTRIES 1

A Final Word 131

Resources 132

Introduction

Imagine you are a man who jumps out of bed in the morning, filled with energy, energized by your dreams, and happy and grateful—regardless of what challenges await. It can be a reality!

My name is Scott Smith, and I've made it my life's focus to wake up rested, enjoy a happy day, sleep peacefully, and repeat. For the longest time, my progress was hit-or-miss. Then, on December 6, 2006, a staggering loss opened my eyes and my heart: I lost my first wife to cancer.

In the months that followed, I worked to make sense of the good and bad of life. I was angry at how something like that could happen to me. But I'm an optimistic guy, so I had to find a way to dig myself out of my hole. One day, I found my shovel when I learned to fill myself with gratefulness for everything that comes my way.

Although my pain didn't go away, my peacefulness returned, and I began to share my new mindset with my *Daily Boost* podcast listeners and coaching clients. That's when I realized many of the men I was working with were feeling similar to the way I once did. I suggested they find something to be grateful for and journal it. And when they did, that's when things began to change for them. The same thing can happen for you. It turns out that the secret to happiness is often found in gratefulness, and gratefulness can be cultivated with a daily journaling practice.

While a journal is a great way to work through complicated feelings, you should consult a professional if you have ongoing or debilitating feelings of depression or anxiety. This book is not a replacement for a therapist, medication, or medical treatment. There is no shame in seeking help.

I didn't have a gratitude journal like this during my journey. I wish I had, but at least I can offer it to you now.

How to Use This Book

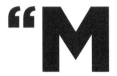

"**M**y life is good. I have a good job. I have a great family, a beautiful home, everything I want. I know I should be grateful . . . but . . . but . . . but . . ."

In my years of coaching, I can't tell you how many men have said those exact words to me. Since most guys are hardwired for the next win and getting down to business, it makes sense. Forget living in the moment! Who has time for that? The problem is that the happiness you seek is found in being grateful, and gratefulness is found in the challenges of your day.

How do you get there?

Slow down—two words I've said to every client I have ever worked with. And now I tell them to you: SLOW DOWN! (Don't worry, it's only for five minutes.)

Ahead of you is a practical, tactical, and gratitude-filled journey designed for your man-mind. Each page has two prompts to encourage you to think, feel, and write; a practice to engage you in what you've been thinking and writing about; and an affirmation that will build gratitude, inspire, and motivate you.

Make a commitment to set aside five minutes every day and complete a single page. An additional notebook may be helpful on your more prolific days. I promise, doing this will not only make your day better, but once you have completed every entry, you will have a personal guide to being happy and grateful that you can reference for the rest of your life.

Your efforts on the coming journey will reveal the sources of feelings and gratefulness in your heart while serving as your trusted guide to living with gratitude every day.

It's time to get started!

WHO MAKES YOU FEEL GRATEFUL?

Who are you grateful for having in your life?

....

....

....

....

How can you express more gratitude to the people you care about most?

....

....

....

....

Between traffic lights, messages, and calls today, allow your mind to fill with images of those who make your life good.

REMINDING MYSELF OF WHY I AM GRATEFUL MAKES ME EVEN MORE UNSTOPPABLE.

LIFE BEGINS WHEN YOU MOVE

What's one recent action that made you feel more grateful about your life?

....

....

....

....

Success begins with one step. What can you do to move forward today?

....

....

....

....

....

Move your body and mind with a gratitude stroll around the neighborhood or a good ol' sweaty workout.

**LIFE IS GREAT WHEN I CHOOSE
TO MOVE TOWARD WHAT I WANT.**

FEELING OPTIMISTIC AND GRATEFUL

What gives you an optimistic feeling about the life you are living?

....

....

....

....

As a man, you may often be encouraged to accept and enjoy a challenge. How do you feel about challenges?

....

....

....

....

Optimistically take on a small, purposeful challenge that, when complete, will make you feel grateful. Keep it small and doable.

WHEN I TAKE ON CHALLENGES WITH OPTIMISM, I FEEL MORE GRATEFUL.

DOING WHAT WORKS BEST FOR YOU

Doing what works best for you leaves no time for what doesn't. What is something that works best for you?

What are you doing when you are at your best? Be specific.

Brainstorm a quick list of what you do best and feel grateful about doing. Set aside time to write down your list in a notebook or journal.

WHEN I FOCUS ON WHAT WORKS BEST FOR ME, I LIVE IN GRATEFULNESS.

YOUR JUKEBOX JOURNEY OF GRATITUDE

Name a few of your favorite artists and songs that make you feel good.

_____

_____

_____

_____

What past musical memories are you grateful for having?

_____

_____

_____

_____

Build a playlist of the songs that have inspired you most in your life. As you listen, think about why each song makes you grateful.

WHEN I LISTEN TO MUSIC THAT INSPIRES ME, I AM MORE GRATEFUL FOR MY JOURNEY.

EMPOWERING YOURSELF TO MOVE FORWARD

What kind of man is your heart telling you that you should be?

....

....

....

....

Describe how grateful you would feel if you were to take action on that message.

....

....

....

....

Before you get busy today, take the time to gratefully do one small thing that your heart is telling you to do.

I AM GRATEFUL WHEN I LISTEN TO MY HEART AND FOLLOW ITS DIRECTIONS.

BECOMING THE MAN YOU'RE MEANT TO BE

What makes you feel good about the man you have become?

....

....

....

....

What would you need to do to become the man you feel you are meant to be?

....

....

....

....

Think about a famous man who inspires you. In your research, pull out a couple of attributes you will implement in your life.

I AM GRATEFUL FOR MY JOURNEY
AND FOR BECOMING THE BEST I CAN BE.

BE SELF-ASSURED, BE NICE

What ways do you feel self-assured that you're grateful for?

....

....

....

....

Whose day will be better today if you are the nicest person they meet?

....

....

....

....

When you find yourself around others today, be self-assured and be nice to someone who isn't expecting it.

WHEN I AM SELF-ASSURED AND NICE TO OTHERS, WE ALL HAVE A NICE DAY.

GRATEFUL TO HAVE TOLD SOMEONE

Who have you recently shared your gratitude with for being present in your life?

_____

_____

_____

_____

Why did you choose to make sure they knew how you felt?

_____

_____

_____

_____

Today, reach out to one person and share why you are grateful for them. In person, phone, text, or email: Choose *their* preferred method.

EVERYONE NEEDS TO KNOW THAT OTHERS ARE GRATEFUL FOR THEM.

A SIMPLE LIFE IS A GOOD LIFE

Being a man in this age can be complicated. In what ways do you wish your life were less complicated?

....

....

....

....

Even a complicated life can be made simpler. What steps can you take to simplify your life?

....

....

....

....

....

Simple is good and often works best. Spend some time and contemplate ways to simplify your life.

WHEN I SIMPLIFY MY LIFE, I AM LIVING A GOOD LIFE.

PROJECTING YOUR FUTURE GRATITUDE

What opportunities are you most excited about in your future?

_____

_____

_____

_____

Why do you, or should you, feel grateful for having them in your life?

_____

_____

_____

_____

We all rise together. Call a friend today to chat about a future that excites both of you.

I AM GRATEFUL FOR EVERY FUTURE OPPORTUNITY I WILL HAVE IN MY LIFE.

THE STORY YOU PRESENT TO THE WORLD

When others think about you, what story are they seeing?

....

....

....

....

If you could change the story, how would it be different?

....

....

....

....

Identify someone you can ask to tell you what they see as the story of your life. Find out if their version matches yours.

WHEN MY ACTIONS MATCH MY STORY, MORE OPPORTUNITIES COME MY WAY.

YOUR FIRST THOUGHT
OF GRATITUDE

What is the first grateful thought that pops into your mind right now?

_____

_____

_____

_____

Why do you suppose that particular thought is the one that came to you?

_____

_____

_____

_____

A simple exercise in gratitude is to take a breath and let three thoughts of gratitude flow from your mind into your journal.

**WHEN I RECOGNIZE A GRATEFUL MOMENT,
I AM LIVING EXACTLY AS I CHOOSE.**

SLOWING DOWN AND LIVING MORE

If you could slow a part of your life down, what would that part be?

....

....

....

....

What if you could slow everything in your life down? How would you do that?

....

....

....

....

Activities that force slowness include yoga, meditation, and even exercise. Purposefully slow down and try one today.

WHEN I SLOW DOWN AND ENJOY THE MOMENT, GRATEFULNESS IS AUTOMATIC.

SMILING WITH GRATITUDE

Imagine yourself outside in the sunlight and feeling grateful.
What are you thinking?

What three people make you smile in gratitude whenever you
think of them?

Greet every person you encounter today with
a big smile while you remember why you are grateful
for them in your life.

I AM A SMILING-WITH-GRATITUDE
MACHINE EVERYWHERE I GO.

YOUR STAIRCASE OF SUCCESS IS WAITING

If success happens one step at a time, what action can you take today?

_____

_____

_____

_____

Climbing higher means looking for the next step. What are the next few steps above you right now?

_____

_____

_____

_____

Pull out your journal and brainstorm the next few steps in your life journey. Don't be shy. Make it big and exciting.

EVERYTHING I WANT IS ACHIEVED ONE STEP AT A TIME.

TIME FOR A GRATITUDE SNEAK ATTACK

Who do you think deserves an unexpected dose of gratitude from you and why?

_____

_____

_____

_____

What is a memorable message you can plan to surprise them with?

_____

_____

_____

_____

Make today the day you surprise someone who really needs it with a gift of gratitude. Be creative and have fun.

I LIVE TO LET OTHERS KNOW HOW GRATEFUL I AM FOR HAVING THEM IN MY LIFE.

EXPLORING YOUR LIFE POSSIBILITIES

When was a time in your life you felt anything was possible?

....

....

....

....

How can you break from your current routine and explore different possibilities today?

....

....

....

....

Keep your notebook near, and when a possibility pops into your mind, write it down. That way it'll be waiting for you when you are ready to act.

WHEN I FEEL STUCK, I CAN STILL AT LEAST IMAGINE POSSIBILITIES.

STOP. THINK. THINK AGAIN. ACT.

Stop, think, think again, and act. What do you need to think about carefully?

_____

_____

_____

_____

After having thought about this, what action do you need to take toward it?

_____

_____

_____

_____

Do you have a favorite place to sit and think? Set aside some thinking time today, and engage in some grateful thought without distraction.

I STOP, THINK, AND THINK AGAIN BEFORE I ACT ON ANYTHING.

THE SIMPLEST WAY
TO SHOW GRATITUDE

Imagine you are sending heartfelt appreciation to someone. Who is it and what are you thanking them for?

....

....

....

....

Keep it simple. One reason I appreciate them in my life is:

....

....

....

....

It doesn't take much time or effort to positively impact someone's day. Send a text message of gratitude and spread the sunshine to the first person who pops into your mind.

IT'S NOT WHAT I SAY TO SOMEONE. IT'S THAT I REMEMBERED TO SAY IT.

EXCITED ABOUT EVERYTHING TO COME

One thing I did as a child that made me feel excited was:

....

....

....

....

One thing I'm looking forward to now that makes me feel excited is:

....

....

....

....

There are 1,440 minutes in a day. Claim thirty of them today to do what excites you. Just imagine how good you will feel.

WHEN I MAKE TIME FOR THINGS THAT ARE EXCITING, MY LIFE FEELS FULLER.

CELEBRATING WHY YOU ARE GRATEFUL

In the last year, what accomplishments made you feel most grateful?

_____

_____

_____

_____

It's easy to gloss over gratefulness. How can you repeat your successful experiences?

_____

_____

_____

_____

Think of one person who has ridden along with you on your journey. Give them a grateful check-in call.

WHEN I'M GRATEFUL FOR MY PAST, I AM GRATEFUL FOR MY FUTURE.

FOCUSING ON WHAT MEANS THE MOST

Distraction is everywhere. Where should you focus instead?

....

....

....

....

Describe the grateful feeling you know you will have after focusing on what means the most.

....

....

....

....

It may be at your desk, in your car, or in nature. Follow your heart to where you focus best and go there today. It's easy if you make the time.

I CAN REACH ANY GOAL WHEN I FOCUS ON WHAT MEANS THE MOST.

MAKING TODAY GREAT FOR SOMEONE

Who could you surprise by uplifting them today?

....

....

....

....

In what small way can you make the day better for everyone you encounter today?

....

....

....

....

Thank-you cards, windshield notes, and even a kind word in the hallway make a day better. Choose one and be a thankful man.

MY BEST DAY HAPPENS WHEN I MAKE SOMEONE ELSE'S DAY.

STAND UP. TAKE A STEP. REPEAT

What goal needs you to stand up, take a step, and get moving?

....

....

....

....

Once you get moving, how do you plan to continue your momentum?

....

....

....

....

Write a book. Start a fitness plan. Grow your relationships. Consider a long-delayed goal and get it moving today.

STAND UP, TAKE A STEP, AND REPEAT. THAT'S ALL I NEED FOR SUCCESS.

SMALL CHANGES MAKE
A GRATEFUL LIFE

What small change can you make in your life that will give you significant results?

....

....

....

....

What significant change in your life will make even your smallest experiences more fulfilling?

....

....

....

....

Make that small change today. Make plans to make a significant change tomorrow.

EVERY POSITIVE CHANGE I MAKE IS LEADING
TO A LIFE I LOVE.

YOUR CHAIN OF SUCCESS KEEPS GOING

Momentum creates a feeling of success. When was the last time you felt personal momentum?

....

....

....

....

What can you do today to continue the success you had yesterday?

....

....

....

....

Take some time today to make a short list of little wins and why they are adding up to a life that you genuinely love.

I WAS MEANT TO MOVE TOWARD SUCCESS, AND I AM GRATEFUL FOR IT.

TOOTING YOUR OWN HORN CAN BE GOOD

Be masculinely egocentric for a moment. What should you be tooting your own horn about?

_____

_____

_____

_____

Who is supportive of you and would revel in your success?

_____

_____

_____

_____

People are waiting to hear your good news.
Choose a place or a way to get in touch, tell them,
and let them celebrate with you.

**WHEN I ALLOW OTHERS TO CELEBRATE MY SUCCESS
WITH ME, I AM GRATEFUL FOR MY LOVED ONES.**

AUTOMATIC, UNSTOPPABLE, NEVER-ENDING MOTIVATION

When was the last time that you felt instantly motivated and why?

....

....

....

....

What can you do to replicate that moment or reason and make yourself feel motivated and unstoppable again?

....

....

....

....

Look for opportunities today that give you
a feeling of being instantly motivated and energized.
Make a note about what works and do it again.

WHEN I PURSUE GOALS THAT MOTIVATE ME FROM INSIDE, LIFE IS MORE FUN.

SPENDING TIME ON THE IMPORTANT

What should you spend more time on and give more attention to in your life?

_____

_____

_____

_____

It is likely that everything on your list seems important, but what deserves real focus?

_____

_____

_____

_____

Use a short meditation to clear your mind of clutter and noise and hear what is important to you. Five minutes is all you need.

WHEN I TAKE TIME FOR WHAT'S IMPORTANT, MY LIFE HAS MORE MEANING.

DOING NOTHING CAN LEAD TO SUCCESS

When did you last do nothing at all and were successful because of it?

....

....

....

....

Describe what doing nothing means to you and how you can do it more often.

....

....

....

....

Today, find a place and do nothing. Use the time to focus on yourself.

WHEN I ALLOW TIME FOR NOTHING, I GET TO DO ANYTHING.

GRATEFULNESS IS ONE DECISION AWAY

As a man who is becoming more attuned to decision-making, what decision can you make that you know will be life-changing?

_____

_____

_____

_____

Now that you know, describe how your life will change because you made the decision.

_____

_____

_____

_____

Make time for a conversation with a friend today and bounce around decisions that will change both of your lives.

THE GRATEFUL AND FULFILLING LIFE I DESIRE IS ONLY ONE DECISION AWAY.

THERE IS ALWAYS
ANOTHER TOMORROW

What didn't you accomplish yesterday that you will prioritize to accomplish today?

_____

_____

_____

_____

If you are caught up on things, what can you do today that fulfills you?

_____

_____

_____

_____

Before your day ends, take a few minutes and pre-plan the essential things you will get done tomorrow, assuring that you will feel more grateful.

EVERY NEW DAY IS MY NEXT OPPORTUNITY TO GROW, THRIVE, AND SUCCEED.

ACCEPTING YOUR TRUE PURPOSE

True purpose in life is found in actions. What do your actions reveal about you?

....

....

....

....

What changes can you make in your actions that will better reveal the real you?

....

....

....

....

What have you been doing instead of living your true purpose? Today, do one thing in alignment with your purpose.

WHEN I CHOOSE TO ACT ON PURPOSE, I LIVE MY PURPOSE.

SELF-INFLICTED SUCCESS FEELS GOOD

You are in charge of your world. What success would you like to create?

_____

_____

_____

_____

Choose an idea that excites you and write the first step that you need to take.

_____

_____

_____

_____

Spend ten minutes today meditating on what it would take for you to alter your entire destiny with your actions. When you finish, write them down.

ALL OF MY SUCCESS IS SELF-INFLICTED. THAT MEANS I CAN DO ANYTHING!

TEACHERS INSPIRE GRATITUDE

Looking back on your life, who was a teacher who had a big impact on you?

....

....

....

....

Now that you are older, what do you appreciate most about them?

....

....

....

....

It feels good to receive gratitude. If possible, consider tracking down a special teacher or mentor and contacting them to share your gratitude.

THE TEACHERS WHO INSPIRED ME IN THE PAST ARE INSPIRING MY FUTURE, TOO.

HOW DO YOU FEEL TODAY?

As a grateful man, how do you want to feel today?
Describe it.

....

....

....

....

What can you do today to create those feelings?

....

....

....

....

Watching a "feel-good" movie is good for the soul.
Choose one and make a plan to watch it this week.
Popcorn is optional.

**I GET TO CHOOSE HOW I FEEL ABOUT EVERYTHING
THAT HAPPENS IN MY LIFE.**

FREE YOUR MIND AND
SET YOURSELF FREE

What is one area of your life where you know you need
a change of mindset?

....

....

....

....

What is the mindset you would like to have in the identified area
of your life?

....

....

....

....

Between activities or tasks today, grab a moment
of mindfulness to shift your mind to the place you
know it should be.

**WHEN I'M MORE MINDFUL OF MY THOUGHTS,
I CONTROL MY FREEDOM.**

IF YOU LEAD, THEY WILL FOLLOW

What vision in your heart requires others to help you succeed?

....

....

....

....

Who would follow you if you stepped up and led with your vision?

....

....

....

....

You'll feel grateful for others helping when you help them, too. Think about people who could use your help.

WHEN I SET THE PATH AND LEAD, OTHERS FOLLOW AND HELP.

DREAMING BIGGER LEADS TO GRATEFULNESS

Living your dreams is where gratefulness begins. What is one dream you have?

....

....

....

....

What can you do today to move closer toward the dream that will make you grateful tomorrow?

....

....

....

....

Big dreamers are all around—and they write books. Search out a book that speaks to your dreams and read a couple of chapters.

WHEN I ACT ON MY DREAMS, I AM EXCITED, HAPPY, AND GRATEFUL.

YOUR PURPOSE IS
FINDING YOUR PURPOSE

What do you think is one purpose to your life?

....

....

....

....

Now list a second and a third.

....

....

....

....

....

The experiences you have today have the power
to draw you closer to your true purpose. Keep an eye
out for those who take you there.

**WHEN MY PURPOSE IS TO FIND MY PURPOSE,
MY HAPPINESS IS INEVITABLE.**

FOLLOWING YOUR PATH TO GRATITUDE

As a man, what daily activities make you feel happy and grateful?

_____

_____

_____

_____

How can you make sure that you have those activities in your life?

_____

_____

_____

_____

Now that you have meaningful activities, pull out your calendar and make sure they are on your path this week.

MY DAILY ACTIVITIES ARE MY PATH TO BEING HAPPY AND GRATEFUL.

WHEN LIFE GETS IN THE WAY

What is your secret for keeping your momentum going no matter what happens?

Translate your secret into three easy steps that you can repeat when needed.

If a difficult moment comes your way today, remember to pause, smile, and use your super powers to keep things moving.

I CAN BUILD MY OWN MOMENTUM.

GRATEFULNESS BEGINS WITH YOUR IDENTITY

As a man, what parts of your personality are you grateful for?

_____

_____

_____

_____

How can you grow to be a more grateful man?

_____

_____

_____

_____

Meditation isn't only for mornings. Extend your lunch by five minutes and meditate on what makes you feel gratitude.

I AM A GRATEFUL PERSON, AND I SHOW IT FROM THE INSIDE OUT.

YOUR BEST LIFE BEGINS TODAY

How would it make you feel if you could start living your dreams today?

What decision could you make right now to move toward that goal?

Review your to-do list, make sure your activities are leading to your best life, and make sure you are doing them today.

MY BEST LIFE BEGINS THE MOMENT I DECIDE THAT IT BEGINS.

CONFIDENT, HAPPY, AND GRATEFUL

When do you feel most confident, happy, and grateful in your life?

....

....

....

....

If you could change anything that would give you even more of that feeling, what would it be?

....

....

....

....

A quick "thank-you" allows you to show—and feel—gratitude. It also builds confidence and happiness. Give a heartfelt "thank-you" to someone today.

I ENJOY BEING A CONFIDENT, HAPPY, AND GRATEFUL MAN.

CHANGING EVERYTHING IN THIRTY DAYS

What goal would you like to accomplish in the next thirty days?

....

....

....

....

What is the first action you will take, and when? Make a plan!

....

....

....

....

Think about a cool place that you can go today that will energize you to sprint toward your goal. Don't work too hard at it. Follow your heart.

I CAN MAKE POSITIVE CHANGES IN MY LIFE IN JUST THIRTY DAYS.

GRATEFUL EVERY
MINUTE OF THE DAY

What thoughts make you feel grateful no matter what else you're going through?

_____

_____

_____

_____

What is a trigger word that will create instant gratitude for you?

_____

_____

_____

_____

Grab a pad of sticky notes and leave yourself positive messages in places that will trigger you to feel more grateful.

NO MATTER WHAT COMES MY WAY, I CAN CONTROL GRATITUDE IN MY LIFE.

YOUR MOMENT
OF YOUR CHANGE

How do you feel about making this moment the time to make
a change? Describe the feeling.

....

....

....

....

Why do you feel the need to make a change?

....

....

....

....

Make a drawing of the change on a piece of
paper. It may not be artistic or even identifiable.
Draw whatever comes to your mind.

**EVERY MINUTE OF THE DAY IS MY POTENTIAL
MOMENT OF CHANGE.**

BEING GRATEFUL FOR YOUR PAST

You are the man you are for a reason. What has gotten you here?

....

....

....

....

How can you turn past lessons into wisdom that guides
your future?

....

....

....

....

Take a moment to send positive energy to someone
you're grateful for having been in your life, wherever
they may be now.

**EVERYTHING I WILL BECOME IN THE FUTURE
IS BECAUSE OF WHO I HAVE BEEN.**

WHAT CAN YOU DO?

What challenges are currently keeping you stuck and would feel
great to remove from your life?

_____

_____

_____

_____

What steps can you take today to remove one or more of
your challenges?

_____

_____

_____

_____

Other men have walked similar paths and can be
a guide to you. Today, spend time exploring people
and groups you can engage for guidance.

**I WILL ALWAYS KEEP MOVING FORWARD WHEN I ASK,
"WHAT CAN I DO?"**

HAPPY AND GRATEFUL IN THE MOMENT

What's something that makes you feel happy and grateful that you haven't yet listed in this journal? Dig deep.

....

....

....

....

What's one more? Dig even deeper.

....

....

....

....

Wherever you go today, see if you can keep yourself in the moment—no matter what happens. Giving a compliment and a smile to others helps.

I AM HAPPY AT THE MOMENT BECAUSE I CHOOSE TO BE HAPPY.

LISTENING TO YOURSELF MORE THAN OTHERS

Your mind is screaming for your attention. What is it saying?

....

....

....

....

What is something you can do today you've been putting off for too long?

....

....

....

....

Find one minute for deep and mindful breathing.
As you do, listen to what your mind is saying to you.

I LISTEN TO WISE PEOPLE, SO I MAKE SURE I LISTEN TO MYSELF.

BELIEVING IN WHO
YOU WILL BECOME

Who do you believe you must become in your life and in
your heart?

....

....

....

....

What are actions you can take to move closer to the best
version of yourself?

....

....

....

....

Sometimes others believe in you more than
you believe in yourself. Reach out to one of those
people today for an uplifting chat.

WHEN I BELIEVE IN MYSELF, I BECOME.
WHEN I BECOME, I ARRIVE.

HOW DO YOU SPEND YOUR TIME?

Time is your most important asset. How do you spend yours wisely?

What activity should you not spend your precious time doing?

There is always time for you to do the important things. Spend your time on the important today, and filter out the rest.

THE WISER I AM ABOUT HOW I USE TIME,
THE MORE GRATEFUL I BECOME.

YOUR EXPECTATIONS LEAD TO GRATITUDE

What recent experience went as you expected and gave you a feeling of gratitude?

_____

_____

_____

_____

What recent experience didn't go as expected, yet you found a way to feel grateful anyway?

_____

_____

_____

_____

If you expect to feel grateful, no matter what happens, you will. Use right now to set your expectations for something coming up in the future.

I ALWAYS FEEL GRATEFUL NO MATTER WHAT HAPPENS IN MY LIFE.

DEEP SENSE OF PERSONAL AWARENESS

What do you think is the personal trait that best describes who you are?

_____

_____

_____

_____

What can you do to amplify that trait in everything you do?

_____

_____

_____

_____

Reach out to a friend who has a deep sense of themself and ask them how they do it.

ANYTHING IS POSSIBLE WHEN I UNDERSTAND WHO I AM ON THE INSIDE.

LIVING IN A POSITIVE
STATE OF MIND

What is one thing in your life you are most positive about?

....

....

....

....

What is one thing in your life you should be more positive about? What steps can you take to do that?

....

....

....

....

Before picking up the phone or entering a meeting, pause to check in with yourself and make sure you are feeling positive.

I STRIVE FOR A POSITIVE MINDSET BECAUSE INSIDE, I AM POSITIVE.

HOLDING SPACE FOR YOUR DREAMS

You are a busy man and today will get busy. What space are you holding for yourself?

When you reclaim your personal space, how will you use it today?

The space between your appointments belongs to you. Find a time today to clear your mind and remember your dreams.

WHEN I HOLD SPACE FOR MY DREAMS, MY DREAMS COME TRUE.

LIVING A LIFESTYLE
OF GRATITUDE

What lifestyle would make you most happy and grateful for being alive?

....

....

....

....

What choices can you make that will allow you to move toward that lifestyle?

....

....

....

....

Make a plan that will enable you to live your chosen lifestyle every day, at least in some small way. There's no need to wait.

I AM GRATEFUL FOR THE LIFESTYLE I HAVE DECIDED TO LIVE.

DON'T BE WHO YOU ARE NOT

What items on your to-do list don't match who you are inside?

How can you drop what isn't you and do more of what is you?

Pay attention to when your heart tells you that something today is not you, and then change your direction.

I LIVE AS MY TRUE SELF. I AM HAPPY, PRODUCTIVE, AND GRATEFUL.

KNOWING YOUR MISSION DRIVES GRATITUDE

Beyond living day-to-day, what is the mission you were born to do?

....

....

....

....

What are you doing every day to drive toward your mission?

....

....

....

....

Research people who are successfully living their mission. Make a few notes about what they are doing well.

KNOWING MY MISSION GIVES ME MORE ENERGY, MOTIVATION, AND PURPOSE.

FREE WILL IS BETTER THAN WILLPOWER

What have you used willpower for that isn't getting done?

_____

_____

_____

_____

Instead of forcing it, what would get you excited to push toward your goals?

_____

_____

_____

_____

Most people use willpower to force themselves. Today, make your first project one that excites you most.

WHEN I DO WHAT EXCITES ME ON THE INSIDE, USING WILLPOWER IS NOT REQUIRED.

FINDING YOUR PURPOSE, LIVING YOUR PASSION

What is something you were passionate about when you were a young boy?

....

....

....

....

How did doing it make you feel? What can you do to replicate that feeling now that you're a man?

....

....

....

....

Today, tap into that feeling you had as a boy, whether by doing the same activity or by doing a new activity that makes you feel that same level of passion.

I ONLY TAKE ACTIONS THAT ARE IN DIRECT ALIGNMENT WITH MY PURPOSE AND PASSION.

SURROUND YOURSELF WITH GRATEFUL PEOPLE

Who are three people you know who seem very grateful?

_____

_____

_____

_____

Would they say that you are grateful? Why or why not?

_____

_____

_____

_____

_____

Success and happiness are a direct result of relationships. Make sure you are surrounding yourself with grateful people today.

WHEN I SURROUND MYSELF WITH GRATEFUL PEOPLE, I AM MORE GRATEFUL.

HOW BADLY DO YOU WANT IT?

What one thing do you want so badly you can't hold
yourself back?

....

....

....

....

How can you turn that exciting thought into today's
real-life experience?

....

....

....

....

....

Build a vision board. Use photos, clippings,
quotes, and more to create a visual representation
of what you want most in your life.

**I CAN DO ANYTHING I DREAM OF IF I WANT IT
BADLY ENOUGH.**

FEELING GREAT MAKING OTHERS FEEL GREAT

If you could make someone feel great today, who would that be?

_____

_____

_____

What secret plan can you spring on them that will make them smile?

_____

_____

_____

Plan and launch a gratitude sneak attack on someone who doesn't expect it but who really deserves it.

WHEN I MAKE OTHERS FEEL GOOD, ALL OF US FEEL GOOD.

ALWAYS LIVING
YOUR AUTHENTIC SELF

When do you feel most authentic, like you are living your true self?

_____

_____

_____

_____

What can you do for yourself today? This isn't about others. This is all about you!

_____

_____

_____

_____

Make time for an activity today that is you being you. Find a way to be your authentic self today.

WHEN I DO ACTIVITIES THAT MAKE ME FEEL LIKE MY TRUE SELF, I BECOME MY TRUE SELF.

MEDITATION ALLOWS TIME FOR GRATEFULNESS

What would stepping off the world for mindful time do for you?

....

....

....

....

If you meditated for fifteen minutes every day, what would you hope to achieve?

....

....

....

....

The time of day doesn't matter. Find fifteen minutes, clear your mind, and let yourself flow into a satisfying meditation session.

WHEN I CLEAR MY MIND AND PAUSE, I FEEL MORE GRATEFUL FOR EVERYTHING.

WHAT DO YOU DO FOR FUN?

Make a list of three things in your life that you do for fun.

....

....

....

....

....

....

How can you integrate those fun things into the next few days?

....

....

....

....

....

Sometimes fun can hide in plain sight, but it leaves clues. Be on the lookout today for anything that makes you smile bigger.

LIFE IS FUN WHEN I MAKE TIME FOR FUN.

GRATITUDE WILL
MAKE YOU SMILE

What about your life gives you a great big smile?

_____

_____

_____

_____

What are ways to integrate more of those "smile moments" into your life today?

_____

_____

_____

_____

Make a point to be receptive to new friends and connections that make your day more enjoyable.

WHEN I SHOW MY GRATITUDE WITH A SMILE, I CAN DO ANYTHING I CHOOSE.

BEING SURE ABOUT YOUR CHOICE

Recall a choice you made that you were grateful for.

_____

_____

_____

_____

Describe the grateful feeling you had when you made that choice.

_____

_____

_____

_____

Spend a few minutes reviewing the choices you are proud of and think about how you can make more good choices in your life.

WHEN I'M PROUD OF MY DECISIONS, I'M PROUD OF MYSELF.

ALWAYS SAYING "YES" TO YOURSELF

When do you say "yes" to yourself?

....

....

....

....

What is one area of life where you should say "yes" to yourself more?

....

....

....

....

Take five minutes to pause and breathe. While you are at it, ask yourself: "What must I do for myself?" Add it to your plan right away.

WHEN I SAY "YES" TO MYSELF, ALL OF MY DREAMS BECOME POSSIBLE.

STATING YOUR GRATEFUL INTENTION

What do you intend to be grateful for having in your life?

....

....

....

....

Your grateful intention will impact others. Who can you influence today?

....

....

....

....

If you want more energy, make a short list of how you intend to be grateful, choose a starting point, and dive in today.

**WHEN I INTEND TO BE MORE GRATEFUL,
I AM MORE GRATEFUL.**

THE TRICK IS THE CLICK

What experience did you have recently that clicked and made you feel grateful?

What can you do to keep those clicks coming today?

A click can be as quick as a millisecond in time. When you get one today, pause, write it down, and savor it. Make it last.

WHEN I GET LIFE CLICKING, I GET THE LIFE THAT I WANT.

YOUR GUT FEELING
IS GUIDING YOU

What is your gut feeling telling you about the life you have built?

....

....

....

....

In what ways has following your gut made your life better?

....

....

....

....

Try to tap into your gut feelings and write down
the small adjustments that you can make for better
insight.

**WHEN I TRUST MY GUT FEELING,
I MAKE GOOD DECISIONS.**

JUMP INTO YOUR DREAMS

What is a long-lost dream of yours that you would love to make a reality?

_____

_____

_____

_____

What action can you take today toward making this dream come true?

_____

_____

_____

_____

Seek out a mentor, in person or online, who has a knack for turning their dreams into reality. Listen to their sage advice.

MY DREAM WILL BECOME REAL WHEN I TAKE A LEAP OF FAITH.

PRE-PLANNED RESPONSES BRING GRATEFULNESS

What is today's significant challenge you'd like to cultivate feelings of gratitude around?

How will you respond to that challenge and make it a grateful day?

Once you've made it through a challenge, remember to feel grateful. Take two minutes to connect to that feeling.

**WHEN I SET AN INTENTION TO FEEL GRATEFUL,
I WILL BE GRATEFUL.**

IF NEXT WEEK NEVER COMES

What is one untaken opportunity presented to you in your life so far that you wish you'd taken?

_____

_____

_____

_____

What is one opportunity in your life so far you are grateful for having taken?

_____

_____

_____

_____

Pull out a pen and paper and doodle your dreams. You know, the ones you should do today in case next week never comes.

OPPORTUNITIES PRESENT THEMSELVES TO ME EVERY DAY.

IT'S YOUR DAY TO FULLY SHOW UP

What relationships do you want to show up for at a higher level?

....

....

....

....

What steps can you take to be fully present for these relationships?

....

....

....

....

Showing up can take many forms, from an email to a conversation. Choose a way and show up to the important moments of your day.

EVERY DAY IS A CHANCE TO SHOW UP AND BE MY TRUE SELF.

SUCCESS FROM MESSY ACTIONS

Perfection is paralyzing. What have you been procrastinating on that you need to get moving?

_____

_____

_____

_____

What less-than-perfect actions can you take to reach your goal?

_____

_____

_____

_____

Today, spend a little time organizing how you plan to attack your goals. When you're ready, get messy. You can clean it up later.

I CAN MAKE PROGRESS TOWARD MY GOALS EVEN BY TAKING MESSY ACTIONS.

WHO IS WAITING FOR YOU?

Who in your life needs you to guide them through a challenge?

....

....

....

....

When it comes to helping others, what gift of wisdom can you give?

....

....

....

....

....

Reach out to someone who needs a kind word, a helping hand, or a smile from you today.

SOMEONE IS WAITING FOR ME TO HAVE A POSITIVE IMPACT ON THEIR LIFE.

BEING GRATEFUL
FOR BEING YOURSELF

What is a quality of your authentic self you haven't yet listed in this journal?

....

....

....

....

What action can you take today to make you grateful to be the man you are?

....

....

....

....

There will be an opportunity for you today to shine and be your authentic self. Your mission is to find it and be it.

I AM GRATEFUL WHEN I AM LIVING MY AUTHENTIC SELF.

BUILDING YOUR BRIDGE TO PASSION

If you were living within your passion, what would you do today?

....

....

....

....

What would need to happen to live within your passion every day?

....

....

....

....

Imagine you need a bridge to get to your passion. Identify the resources to build the bridge to where you are going in your life.

EVERYTHING I DO TODAY IS ABOUT BUILDING A BRIDGE TO MY FUTURE.

GRATITUDE IN THE BODY

What's one aspect of your health that you're grateful for?

....

....

....

....

Dig deep and list two more aspects of your health and/or body that you are grateful for.

....

....

....

....

Engage in some healthy body movement today. Hold your chin high, think of the people who make you smile, and move or stretch in your preferred way!

MY BODY SUPPORTS ME, AND I SUPPORT MY BODY.

WAVING YOUR MAGIC WAND

If you had a magic wand, what would you instantly make happen in your life?

Now that you know what you want, what realistic steps will make it happen?

As you go about living today, when you notice a little goodness happen (the wand being waved), say "Thank you!" to the universe.

LIFE IS MAGICAL. I AM THE BEST MAGICIAN IN THE WORLD.

CONSISTENT ACTIONS EQUAL CONSISTENT SUCCESS

What is consistently working for you in your journey to success?

How can you continue your progress and feel grateful for doing it?

Sometimes it isn't easy to see your success.
Ask a buddy what they think works best for you,
and listen to them.

WHEN I REPEAT WHAT WORKS FOR ME, GRATITUDE IS INEVITABLE.

YOU NEED A REMINDER TO RECHARGE

Is it time to take some kind of break in your life? Why or why not?

_____

_____

_____

_____

What recharges you the most?

_____

_____

_____

_____

Somewhere nearby, there is a place that provides you an injection of good energy. Go there today.

I AM ALWAYS MORE GRATEFUL WHEN I TAKE THE TIME TO RECHARGE MYSELF.

YOUR DEFINITION OF GRATITUDE IS EVERYTHING

In your gratitude journey, what does being grateful now mean to you?

....

....

....

....

What new ways can you cultivate that new meaning?

....

....

....

....

A great way to feel instant gratitude is by building a video playlist of short, inspiring clips that you can turn on at any time. Set aside time to do that today.

WHEN I DEFINE MY FEELING OF GRATITUDE, I CAN CREATE MORE IN MY LIFE.

SOMETIMES IT'S BEST TO SAY NOTHING

Is there a situation you're in that's better served by saying nothing?

....

....

....

....

How will you respond instead of speaking? With a smile? With a nod? Or with nothing at all?

....

....

....

....

Think about how much more smoothly some things can go when you hold back, allow time to reflect, and respond. Pause before you act today.

MY BEST RESPONSE IS SOMETIMES NO RESPONSE AT ALL—AND IT FEELS GOOD.

GRATEFUL FOR
EVERYTHING YOU HAVE

What's one thing you're grateful for that might surprise others?

_____

_____

_____

_____

What challenges have you been through that gave you an unexpectedly grateful feeling?

_____

_____

_____

_____

Search around today, in person or online, and find someone who is going through an unimaginable challenge or tragedy, and yet they remain grateful.

TODAY, I AM GRATEFUL FOR EVERYTHING THAT CROSSES MY LIFE PATH.

IS IT TIME TO STEP UP YOUR GAME?

What does stepping up your game mean to you?

....

....

....

....

What is one area where you know you can step up your game?

....

....

....

....

Meet with someone who has your best interest in mind and ask them for suggestions on how you can step up your game.

WHEN I STEP UP MY GAME, I SHINE BRIGHTER AND AM HAPPIER.

NEVER WEAR YOURSELF OUT AGAIN

What in your life is draining you of energy and needs to be moved out of your life?

_____

_____

_____

_____

Life is full of energy-draining things. List two more that need to go.

_____

_____

_____

_____

What's the most energy-infusing thing you do? Spend a few minutes doing that today.

I AM GRATEFUL TO FOCUS ON WHAT GIVES ME ENERGY AND GRATEFULNESS.

CHANGE YOUR STORY, CHANGE YOUR LIFE

If you could change your story, what would the new version be?

_____

_____

_____

_____

List three ways that you can rewrite the story of your life.

_____

_____

_____

_____

Visit or chat with someone who can give you guidance on how to live a life of never-ending gratitude.

MY STORY EVOLVES, AND TODAY'S LESSONS WILL MAKE ME STRONGER THAN EVER.

PAUSE FOR GRATEFULNESS

What do you need to pause in your life so that you can feel more gratitude?

_____

_____

_____

_____

Who do you need to pause in your life so that you can feel more gratitude?

_____

_____

_____

_____

Pause and take a mind-clearing break today. Think about what makes you feel grateful and what doesn't.

I FEEL MORE GRATITUDE WHEN I PAUSE AND THINK ABOUT MORE GRATITUDE.

THE MONKEY IN THE MIDDLE

Are you feeling stuck in the middle? What has you stuck?

_____

_____

_____

_____

Empower yourself by choosing a direction. What direction will you go? What will power you?

_____

_____

_____

_____

Reflect on a time you were stuck in the middle and broke out.

I CHOOSE TO BREAK OUT OF THE MIDDLE AND WIN.

ACHIEVING YOUR GOALS
AND FEELING GRATEFUL

What is the most vital skill you use to succeed on a daily basis?

How can you better use that skill to feel more grateful today
and every day?

Look for ways to use your unique talents and mindset
in everything you do today.

WHEN I FOCUS ON MY STRENGTHS, I FEEL GOOD
ABOUT MYSELF AND MY WORK.

FEWER CHOICES
ARE YOUR FRIEND

What distracting choices can you eliminate to attain what you desire more quickly?

By focusing on what is important, life becomes more fulfilling. So, what's important to you?

Experiencing a simpler world will inspire you. Spend some quiet time in nature today, gathering your thoughts.

MY TRUE FREEDOM IS FOUND WITH FEWER CHOICES AND BY FOCUSING ON WHAT'S IMPORTANT.

GRATEFUL FOR THINGS, TOO

What's one inanimate thing you're grateful for? Why are you grateful for it?

....

....

....

....

What are two more, and why are you grateful for them?

....

....

....

....

Recommend one of these things to a friend today—or even a stranger.

I FIND GRATITUDE IN ALL FORMS IN MY LIFE.

LIVING MORE BY DOING LESS

Before you start your day, what task can you responsibly eliminate?

....

....

....

....

When your chore list is shortened, you have more time to do what you love. What do you love to do?

....

....

....

....

Today, rework your schedule and alternate doing more with breaks of doing less.

WHEN I DON'T FILL EVERY MINUTE OF THE DAY, I HAVE HOURS FOR MYSELF!

A GOOD LIFE IS FILLED WITH GRATITUDE

No matter how crazy today is, what will you be grateful for?

_____

_____

_____

_____

Who are you grateful for today, and how can you show them?

_____

_____

_____

_____

Choose one person in your life, reach out, and make sure they know you are grateful for them.

WHEN I APPROACH EVERY DAY AS A GRATEFUL DAY, EVERY DAY IS BETTER.

BEING A GOOD QUITTER
FEELS GOOD

What are you doing that needs to come to an end soon?

....

....

....

....

If you gave it up, what goodness would you replace it with?

....

....

....

....

Instead of doing something you'd rather not do, spend your focus today on ending what isn't serving you and beginning what does.

WHEN I AM A GOOD QUITTER, I AM FOCUSING ON WHAT'S IMPORTANT.

ALWAYS DOING
THE RIGHT THING

When your behavior aligns with your values, you are living in gratitude. What is one of your values?

_____

_____

_____

_____

What is a behavior you can align to this value?

_____

_____

_____

_____

Review your to-do list and decide how you will do the right thing for everyone involved—including yourself.

I AM GRATEFUL TO BE A MAN WHO ASPIRES TO DO THE RIGHT THING.

EXPANDING YOUR COMFORT ZONE

You will feel grateful when you are growing as a person. What activities make you feel that way?

_____

_____

_____

_____

Expanding your comfort zone is better than stepping out of it. How can you expand it?

_____

_____

_____

_____

Try something that expands your comfort zone: Join a fitness class. Journal more. Learn a few words of a new language.

WHEN I COMFORTABLY EXPAND MY COMFORT ZONE, I ENJOY WHAT I DO MORE.

TELLING THE STORY OF YOU

What story is living within you that makes you
utterly unique?

....

....

....

....

How can you tell your story so others better understand you?

....

....

....

....

Sometimes it helps when you ask others how they
see you as a person. Find someone you respect—and
listen to them.

**WHEN I LIVE MY UNIQUE STORY, I AM HAPPIER
AND MORE GRATEFUL.**

IT'S A
GOING-WITH-THE-FLOW DAY

What inspiring thought is wandering in your mind that would
benefit from action?

....

....

....

....

Instead of resisting, how can you move forward with gratitude
and thanks?

....

....

....

....

Today is a going-with-the-flow kind of day.
As your day unfolds, hold on to going with the flow
with gratitude.

**WHEN I LET MY INSPIRATION FLOW WITHOUT
INTERRUPTION, MY LIFE FLOWS, TOO.**

BRING OUT YOUR INNER FIVE-YEAR-OLD

If you were five years old, what would you be doing right now?

_____

_____

_____

_____

Think about what fascinated you as a child. Does any of it still fascinate you?

_____

_____

_____

_____

Why not let yourself be a big kid for a moment?
Forget adulting; inspiration is everywhere.
Get curious and go find it!

**WHEN I LOOK AT THE WORLD AS A CHILD,
LIFE IS FULL OF WONDER.**

EVERYTHING YOU WANT STARTS HERE

No matter how big your dream, it starts where you are.
What needs to start?

Decide on your first step toward making your dream a reality.
How can you build momentum?

Feel excited about making your fantastic future real
and commit to starting today. One small step is all
it takes.

**NO MATTER WHERE I AM IN LIFE,
MY FUTURE STARTS HERE.**

ONLY YOUR PERMISSION IS REQUIRED

What is something you have been waiting for someone's permission to do?

_____

_____

_____

_____

What is something you can give yourself permission to do today?

_____

_____

_____

_____

Dig out your old list of goals (or try to remember them), choose one, and give yourself permission to begin. Your permission is what matters.

THE ONLY PERMISSION I NEED TO BE HAPPY IS THE PERMISSION I GIVE MYSELF.

MANAGING THE WINDS OF LIFE

The blowing winds of life lead to many places. Where have they carried you?

....

....

....

....

If the winds are blowing you off course, how can you adjust today?

....

....

....

....

Seek advice from others on how you can harness the winds of life and move toward your goals.

THE WINDS OF LIFE WILL CARRY ME WHEREVER I CHOOSE TO GO.

EVERY DAY IS A DO-OVER DAY

What life experience would you like a retry at, in order to build your best life?

....

....

....

....

Why would you do it again? What outcome would you expect this time around?

....

....

....

....

Meditation is great for reflecting on how you can improve in the future and attain better results. Five minutes should do it.

EVERY DAY IS MY CHANCE TO MAKE TODAY EVEN BETTER THAN THE ONE BEFORE.

HOW TO BECOME
YOUR DREAM YOU

Who would you be if you loved yourself more?

....

....

....

....

In what ways can you adjust your day to make
it more you?

....

....

....

....

Put on the album you find most inspiring, feel the
good vibes, and let your mind wander to the person
you want to become.

**WHEN I KNOW WHO I DREAM OF BECOMING,
I BECOME.**

TODAY'S CHALLENGES
ARE OPPORTUNITIES

Challenges are opportunities to grow. What are today's biggest challenges?

....

....

....

....

How will you use your challenging experiences to grow and be more grateful?

....

....

....

....

Today, search out opportunities that, though they may be challenging, will give you what you want on the other side.

I SEEK CHALLENGES IN LIFE BECAUSE THERE
IS AN OPPORTUNITY ON THE OTHER SIDE.

TODAY'S CHALLENGES GIVE TOMORROW'S GRATEFULNESS

What's one challenge you have faced that has made you more grateful?

....

....

....

....

How have you been rewarded and become grateful because of the experience?

....

....

....

....

Choose one challenge in your life and take a small step toward facing it.

WHEN I EMBRACE TODAY'S CHALLENGES, I WILL BE MORE GRATEFUL TOMORROW.

HOW TO GET LUCKY IN LIFE

Luck is a result of preparation. What are you preparing for?

....

....

....

....

What do you need to do to ensure you have luck when you need it?

....

....

....

....

....

Review your goals and dream list and make sure you are preparing for your ultimate success.

I GET LUCKY IN LIFE WHEN I AM PREPARED
FOR MY LIFE.

FIRING UP YOUR ANTICIPATION ENGINE

What future event gets you so excited that you feel like a child?

....

....

....

....

What is an event that fires you up that you can add to your "adult" calendar?

....

....

....

....

Fire up your Anticipation Engine and make a plan that gets you excited about tomorrow.

WHEN I HAVE SOMETHING TO LOOK FORWARD TO, LIFE IS MORE FUN.

YOUR DREAMS DESERVE
YOUR ATTENTION

What dream project deserves your attention today?

_____

_____

_____

_____

What consistent and small actions could you do to move this
dream project forward?

_____

_____

_____

_____

Set aside time to pick up a long-lost and important
project. Invest a few minutes to breathe life
into it again.

**WHEN I TAKE SMALL AND FOCUSED ACTION,
EVERYTHING IN LIFE IS EASIER.**

FEELING LIKE THE UNDERDOG

Recall a time when you felt empowered, in control, successful, and happy.

....

....

....

....

Now recall a time when you felt the opposite—like you were the underdog.

....

....

....

....

....

Look for an opportunity to help someone who feels like the underdog today. You'll automatically feel like a superstar.

EVEN WHEN I FEEL LIKE THE UNDERDOG, I CAN STILL COME OUT ON TOP.

PATTING YOURSELF ON THE BACK

In the past week, what accomplishments made you feel the proudest?

....

....

....

....

Recognizing when you do well feels great. How can you do more of that for yourself?

....

....

....

....

Find a quiet spot, reach over your shoulder, and pat yourself on the back. You deserve it. Do it several times for maximum impact.

WHEN I CELEBRATE MY SUCCESS, I KNOW MORE IS ON THE WAY.

CONNECTING IS BETTER
THAN COLLECTING

Who can you reach out to and develop a more meaningful
relationship with?

_____

_____

_____

_____

Who can you begin a *new* and rewarding relationship
with today?

_____

_____

_____

_____

Collecting names and networking mindlessly
isn't always rewarding for your soul. Pay attention
and find meaning in your relationships today.

**WHEN I CONNECT DEEPLY WITH OTHERS,
EVERYONE IS SERVED AT A HIGHER LEVEL.**

YOUR SOMEDAY
HAS ARRIVED TODAY

What have you been waiting for that you will make happen today?

....

....

....

....

You'll love yourself when you focus on your dreams. What is your biggest dream?

....

....

....

....

You may be waiting for someday to arrive. There's no need to wait. Do what you've been putting off.

**WHEN I CHOOSE TO MAKE IT HAPPEN,
THE SOMEDAY I AM WAITING FOR IS TODAY.**

YOUR REWARD FOR HARD
WORK IS OPPORTUNITY

Working hard at what you love is called passion. What is your
passion?

....

....

....

....

How can you do what you love, get paid more, and feel
gratitude?

....

....

....

....

Journal and brainstorm the kind of work that you
can do until you don't want to work anymore.

**MY REWARD FOR DOING WELL IS ANOTHER CHANCE
TO DO EVEN MORE.**

YOUR VALUES DRIVE YOUR LIFE

Personal values guide your life. What are your three guiding values lately?

_____

_____

_____

_____

How can you make sure that you are living your guiding values today?

_____

_____

_____

_____

Find a way to live out each of your guiding values today. Infuse them into your activities and interactions.

WHEN I LIVE MY GUIDING VALUES, I AM LIVING MY BEST LIFE.

RECEIVING AND BEING
A POSITIVE INFLUENCE

Who or what is a positive influence that you feel grateful to have in your life?

How does that person or thing help you be the man you want to be?

In everything you do today, commit to being a positive influence for whomever you meet.

I ALWAYS SEEK POSITIVE INFLUENCES,
AND I AM A POSITIVE INFLUENCE.

CHOOSING TO THRIVE EVERY DAY

What thoughts give you a feeling of being alive, growing, and thriving?

_____

_____

_____

_____

How can you apply those thoughts to challenging moments and continue thriving?

_____

_____

_____

_____

Listen to yourself, trust your thoughts, and take action on them. Happiness is yours for the taking.

WHEN I LISTEN TO MYSELF, I LIVE, GROW, AND THRIVE.

ARE YOU KEEPING YOUR VISION?

What vision in your mind makes you feel excited and grateful?

....

....

....

....

How can you keep that vision alive in your life every day?

....

....

....

....

On paper, a computer, or a whiteboard, brainstorm the vision that you hold within yourself—and start living it.

WHEN I HAVE A VISION FOR WHAT I WANT MOST, I GET WHAT I WANT MOST.

WAKING UP DAILY
WITH GRATITUDE

What would you like your grateful thoughts to be every morning?

....

....

....

....

If you prioritized the order of your grateful thoughts, what's most important?

....

....

....

....

Going to sleep quickly and waking up slowly makes for good dreams and great days. Take your time tomorrow morning.

BEFORE I AM ANYTHING, I AM GRATEFUL
FOR EVERYTHING IN MY LIFE.

LIVING IS ABOUT YOUR EXPERIENCE

What life-changing experiences are you dreaming of bringing into your life?

....

....

....

....

You'll feel grateful for following your dreams. How can you begin today?

....

....

....

....

Go old-school: Visit a bookstore, wander the shelves, and be inspired by the experiences of others that magically jump off the shelves.

I MAKE EVERY EXPERIENCE THE BEST EXPERIENCE IT CAN BE.

FOCUSING ON WHAT'S IMPORTANT

What are the most critical aspects of your life to focus on?

....

....

....

....

What distracting items can you remove from your to-do list so you can focus?

....

....

....

....

Ask a friend or loved one what they think is distracting you. Then take steps to reduce or eliminate the distraction.

I AM GRATEFUL WHEN I TAKE TIME TO FOCUS ON WHAT IS IMPORTANT.

DOING WHAT MAKES
YOUR HEART SING

What are you doing when you live in the moment?

....

....

....

....

Doing what you love, loving every minute. What's one thing you love to do that you haven't listed yet?

....

....

....

....

Whether you love museums, fishing, playing golf, or just hanging out, trust your gut and do what makes your heart sing today.

**WHEN I DO WHAT MAKES MY HEART SING,
I AM HAPPY AND GRATEFUL.**

A FINAL WORD

Congratulations on completing the journal you hold in your hands. I hope it gives you a sense of accomplishment, pride, and gratefulness.

With your dedication, the pages of your competed journal will serve as a reference guide for feeling grateful in your life for years to come. Be sure to keep it handy and implement what you have discovered about yourself in daily action.

As you learned through this process, living with a sense of gratitude is found in your daily challenges, good and bad. Being mindful of those situations makes for a much more satisfying life. You'll be happier, content, and excited about what is to come, and others will notice the changes. In short, gratitude will make for a much more joyful life.

In closing, I encourage you to continue to explore gratitude and practice gratitude journaling through your life. There is no better way to feel a sense of purpose and passion than by being grateful for whatever the world brings you.

Resources

***Daily Boost* Podcast**
The inspirations for this book were initially explored and continue to play out on my *Daily Boost* podcast. Listen and follow at DailyBoostPodcast.com/follow

MotivationToMove.com
Master life's challenges every day while building a happy and successful life at MotivationToMove.com

Face your passion at FaceYourPassion.com

Follow the man who ran across America at CroixSather.com

Tom Beal is a Marine who obsessively focuses on "making today great" at TheSimplifier.com

Find your inspiration to create a better life with NinaAmir.com

Troy Broussard is a former Navy nuclear sub crew member with thousands of life hacks at TroyBroussard.com/gratitude

Acknowledgments

This book would not be possible without the positive influence of others in my life.

My mother is a shining example of living a joyful and positive life. She passed that on to me.

My late wife, Sheryl, encouraged me to do what makes my heart sing, and I have. After she passed, Joi entered my life, bringing her endlessly "joyful" personality.

My daughter Carlyn's and my son Austin's enthusiasm and support have been more than any dad could ask for.

Lastly, thank you to my listeners, clients, friends, and mentors, who have all played a role in the strategies you have experienced in this book.

About the Author

 Scott Smith is the Chief Motivation Officer of MotivationToMove.com and the host of the *Daily Boost* podcast, which—with over 50 million downloads—is one of the top 500 podcasts globally.

A lifelong communicator, Scott has spoken on stages around the world and across various types of media, taught courses and conducted training, and works regularly with clients in groups and individually.

Scott focuses on helping you find your purpose by doing what makes your heart sing and following his simple recipe for success: Stand up, take a step, *repeat* . . . until you get what you want.

CPSIA information can be obtained
at www.ICGtesting.com
Printed in the USA
BVHW021959130922
646926BV00022B/549